GLUTEN FREE AND HAPPY

Danielle Elliott

Contents

Introduction	iv
Dedication	vii
Disclaimer	viii

CHAPTER 1:
Coeliac disease vs. Non-coeliac gluten sensitivity — 1

CHAPTER 2:
Why the apparent increase in sensitivity? — 11

CHAPTER 3:
What actually happens in Coeliac disease? — 15

CHAPTER 4:
What if your symptoms continue? — 18

CHAPTER 5:
Why a gluten free diet may not be enough — 24

CHAPTER 6:
Associated medical conditions — 31

CHAPTER 7:
Improving your digestive health & what to do during acute attacks — 35

CHAPTER 8:
The heart of the home - the kitchen   40

CHAPTER 9:
Bringing happy back   43

CHAPTER 10 :
Gluten free diet in children & teens   50

CHAPTER 11:
Your everyday living resource   53

CHAPTER 12:
Recipes   69

INTRODUCTION

For many of us the way our digestive system works to breakdown and digest our food, and produce waste, happens all on its own. It is something we don't need to think about or concentrate on. That is until things get uncomfortable or even painful. Even then, some people go for years ignoring what is happening on the inside, hoping it will just go away.

The truth is that our gut does a lot more than digest and absorb food and make waste. It is a huge and complex system that interacts with all areas of our body. The gut is not just the digestive system, it is also a sense organ (thus where we get our "gut feeling" from) and a huge part of our immune system. It has more nerves than the rest of the peripheral nervous system and makes more decisions in a day about our immunity, than the rest of the immune system does in a lifetime. It is the first point of contact with food, foreign particles, bacteria and viruses, for our internal system.

No wonder it can be the starting point for much inflammation and many diseases. Coeliac disease (**CD**) and Non coeliac gluten sensitivity (**NCGS**) make it necessary to follow a gluten free (**GF**) diet. With this comes a huge change to your everyday diet and lifestyle. It affects every area of your life, as we generally eat something substantial 3-5 times a day, plus all the incidental things we put into our mouths without realising, for example, if someone offers us a chip or a lolly.

Food has the power to make us happy and at times to make us unwell. There is so much joy that can come from food and sharing it with others. When you are diagnosed with CD or NCGS, it can feel like that is over and that you will never enjoy food again or possibly feel the same happiness. It is a huge thing to take on and there is a lot of grief and loss that you may need to work through. For some there is also huge relief, as they finally know why they have been suffering, especially if it has taken years for a diagnosis.

I have written this book, as I wanted to share all that we have learned since my husband was diagnosed with CD. I realised how much we have learned in four years and how this has just become second nature to us. Initially becoming GF seemed so daunting, despite the fact that I am a naturopath, there was still a lot to learn. I believe knowledge and understanding can give you huge amounts of power. When you are first diagnosed you can feel like that has been taken away, but as you learn what you can do and have, not just what you are missing out on, I feel you can regain power and control. I believe this can help to make you happy again. None of us like having control over our life taken away.

In this book you will find all of the background information on symptoms, diagnosis and options you have if your symptoms continue, while strictly following a

GF diet. The physical changes that happen in CD and NCGS are covered as are suggestions on what you can do to improve your digestive health, speed up recovery and tips on what to do during an acute attack are also included. I also review the emotional impact this diagnosis may have and suggest ideas on making home life, eating out and travelling both safe and pleasurable. There are also some recipes to bring joy back into the foods you may be missing and a huge resource section to help you shop and read labels safely.

I hope that reading this book brings more knowledge, joy and happiness into your life.

DEDICATION

This book is dedicated to all of those living and working with CD and gluten sensitivity. It can sometimes feel like you are such a small group or that you are on your own, but I have learned that there are so many out there helping others and wanting to learn – this book is for you.

Thank you to all of the people who have provided me with resources and information to make this book complete.

Also, a big thank you to my husband, for giving me the time and space to write this book. Without you and all that we have learned on this journey together, this book would not exist.

DISCLAIMER

This book is not intended as a substitute for the medical advice of your GP or specialist or any other health professional. The reader should regularly consult a health practitioner, in matters relating to his/her health and particularly with respect to any symptoms that may require diagnosis or medical attention. The information contained in this book is based on my personal and naturopathic clinical experiences. It does not apply to everyone's situation. It is my intention that the information in this book be helpful and supportive in your quest to be GF and happy.

If you believe you may have coeliac disease or non-coeliac gluten sensitivity, then you should see your GP for proper testing and diagnosis.

Chapter 1

COELIAC DISEASE vs NON-COELIAC GLUTEN SENSITIVITY

Coeliac disease affects the tissue of the small intestine, this is the area that has the function of absorbing the nutrients from the foods we have eaten. When someone has coeliac disease and this tissue comes into contact with gliadin (one of the two proteins that make up gluten), it starts an immune reaction. This reaction ultimately destroys the lining of the small intestine, making it very difficult for it to do its job, including the absorption of nutrients. The figures show that it affects about 1% of the population in western countries. But some researchers believe the figure would actually be about 5%, because there are so many people living with the condition, undiagnosed.

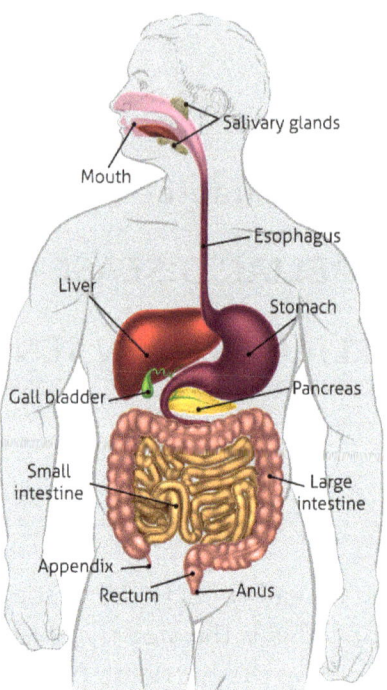

Our food moves from our mouth to our stomach and then makes its way to the small intestine which is where gluten reacts with the immune system in CD and where the damage to the lining takes place.

Gliadin is found in gluten, which is a protein in wheat, rye, barley and triticale (a cereal crop developed from crossing wheat and rye). Oats contain a protein very similar to gluten and so must be avoided too. Any food made from part of these foods need to be avoided too. A comprehensive list can be found in the Everyday Living Resource section of this book on page 53.

The damage to the tissue is reversed once a completely

GF diet is adopted. This repair is a very lengthy process, it has even been found to take up to several years. Natural medicine can help to support the repair of the small intestine and possibly help to improve symptoms quicker.

Coeliac disease can develop at any age, even if you have been able to eat wheat in the past with no side-effects. It is an auto-immune condition. An auto-immune condition develops when your body starts seeing normally safe foods, particles or cells as foreign and something that needs to be attacked. In the case of coeliac disease your body starts to view gluten and the cells in your small intestine, as things that will hurt you and so it mounts an immune response, which ultimately destroys the lining of the small intestine. There are many auto-immune conditions and they attack different cells in the body. Another example is Type I Diabetes, where the body starts to see the cells that make insulin (Islet cells found in the pancreas) as the enemy and destroys them. This leads to the person not being able to make insulin and therefore needing to rely on insulin injections to maintain healthy blood sugar levels.

Non-coeliac gluten sensitivity (NCGS) is thought to affect 6% of the population, and has only recently gained more scientific validation of its existence. It has been debated in scientific journals since about 1980. Today though more and more people are choosing to eat GF, even though they have been told they do not have CD. This is because they have noticed that their symptoms improve while following a GF diet. This change has driven the availability of GF foods in supermarkets and when eating out. This is great news for everyone who needs to exclude gluten containing foods from their eating plan.

NCGS it is not an autoimmune reaction or an allergic one, this means their body in not mounting an immune reaction. The cells in the small intestine look normal and there is no scarring but there are definite symptoms in the person when they consume gluten. These symptoms improve on a gluten free diet.

The latest research is showing the possibility of inflammation markers being present. However, it is too early at this stage for definitive testing.

SYMPTOMS

The symptoms of CD can vary immensely between people. Some people experience severe symptoms while others have no obvious symptoms. Symptoms can include one or more of the following:

- Gastrointestinal symptoms including diarrhoea, constipation, nausea, vomiting, flatulence, cramping, bloating, abdominal pain, stetorrhea (fatty stool)

- fatigue, weakness and lethargy

- iron deficiency anaemia and/or other vitamin and mineral deficiencies

- failure to thrive or delayed puberty in children

- weight loss (although some people may gain weight)

- bone and joint pains or osteoporosis

- recurrent mouth ulcers and/or swelling of mouth or tongue

- altered mental alertness, depression and irritability

- skin rashes such as dermatitis herpetiformis

- bruising easily

Please know that some people are symptom free too.

People who experience any of the following should also be screened for CD:

- early onset osteoporosis
- unexplained infertility and miscarriage
- family history of CD
- liver disease
- autoimmune disease including type 1 diabetes, autoimmune thyroid conditions

Comparing symptoms of coeliac disease and non-coeliac gluten sensitivity

COELIAC DISEASE	NON COELIAC GLUTEN SENSITIVITY
Fatigue	Fatigue
Weight loss	Headache
Diarrhoea	Diarrhoea
Anaemia	Anaemia
Osteoporosis	Joint pain
Depression	Foggy brain

Dermatitis herpetiformis (a blistering skin rash that is linked with CD)	Eczema/rash
Tingling, numbness and/or pain in the hands and feet	Numbness in legs/arms/fingers
	Abdominal pain/IBS symptoms
	History of food allergy in infancy

Diagnosis of coeliac disease usually starts with a referral for some blood tests (as described below in Testing Available). This can come from your GP, specialist or natural healthcare practitioner. If someone is eating a diet containing gluten and has coeliac disease they will test positive to antibodies for gliadin (the protein found in gluten) and self (their own tissue, as this is an autoimmune condition). When these two tests come back positive a gastroenterologist will then usually confirm the diagnosis by performing an endoscopy. To look at the small bowel for tissue damage and take a small biopsy (a small amount of tissue). It is a day procedure performed under a light anaesthetic. Biopsies need to be taken, as in some individuals the tissue damage may not be seen by the naked eye (or camera used in the procedure).

If you are already on a GF diet and testing is done

then you may get a false negative test result. So it is important to not be on a GF diet prior to testing. If you have been on a GF diet for a while, a diet including gluten would need to be resumed for at least six weeks prior to testing as per the guidance from your specialist. The recommendation from "Coeliac Australia" is that for testing to be accurate, an adult must consume the equivalent of 4 slices of wheat bread per day and 2 slices for children per day. They say that although you may be worried about severe symptoms during this gluten challenge period, the symptoms usually reduce over time due to the damage to the small intestine lining.

It is very important to get testing done accurately and have a clear and reliable diagnosis for the future of your health. If you get a false negative, you may feel you are able to include small amounts of gluten in your diet and if you do have CD you will continue to damage your gut lining. Some other really important reasons to be diagnosed correctly are:

- To have the support of your doctor or gastroenterologist and /or dietician throughout your life

- To be sure that a 100% GF diet is absolutely essential for life

- To minimise the health complications of not adhering to a GF diet in CD

- In children, it is essential to allow for their best growth and development

- To inform first degree relatives, so that they too can be tested for CD

TESTING AVAILABLE

IgA tissue trans-glutaminase antibodies (IgA TTG Abs) – This test is very sensitive and accurate as long as the person has eaten gluten leading up to testing. Otherwise the immune system may not be stimulated and there could be a false negative.

IgG deaminated gliadin peptide antibodies (IgG DGP Abs) – The presence of deaminated gliadin is found only in coeliac patients, so is the recommended test. This test also requires the person to have consumed gluten leading up to the test for it to be accurate.

Genetic testing for CD – There are two genes involved in CD that we know of. Up to 97% of patients with CD have one of these genes, if not both (HLA-DQ2 and HLA – DQ8). Just because you have one of these genes, does not mean that you will have CD in your lifetime, there is still a need for something to trigger these genes to express. About 30% of the population has one or both of these genes and of these people about 3% will end up living with CD.

If someone in your family has a positive test result for CD then all immediate family members should also be screened for a couple of reasons. One is that not all people with CD have symptoms, it is thought that 4 out of 5 people with CD are undiagnosed. Another reason is that leaving CD untreated can lead to many other complications including other severe autoimmune conditions, like thyroid disease and type 1 diabetes.

If your specialist suspects CD and some of your blood

tests have been negative, they may choose to do the genetic testing. If you do have one or both of the genes, it does not necessarily indicate you have CD presently. This testing is more useful to rule out CD, when the results come back and say the genes are not present. It can also give peace of mind to parents, who themselves have CD. If your child is suffering with tummy symptoms and they test negative to the genes, then you can be reassured it is not CD and with the information we have today, you can be assured they will not develop it later in life.

Diagnosis of non-coeliac gluten sensitivity is similar to the diagnosis of IBS (Irritable Bowel Syndrome). It is a diagnosis of exclusion. So we would say someone has NCGS when their other tests for coeliac and wheat allergy come back negative and they have improvement of their symptoms once they exclude gluten from their diet. So someone who has negative tests results for the TTG and DGP antibodies may be tested for anti-gliadin antibodies. This test is positive in around 50% of people with NCGS, so can help to support the person's observations. This was one of the early tests for coeliac disease, but was replaced by the two other tests as it was not found to be positive in 100% of patients with CD.

Interpreting tests results for Coeliac disease

IgA TTG Abs	IgG DGP Abs	HLA genes	Interpretation
+	+	+	Coeliac disease
+	+	-	Coeliac disease
-	+	+	Most likely coeliac disease
-	+	-	Most likely coeliac disease
+	-	+	Most likely coeliac disease
+	-	-	Most likely coeliac disease
-	-	-	Not coeliac disease, test anti-gliadin antibody
-	-	+	Unlikely coeliac, but check gluten ingestion prior to testing

Chapter 2

WHY THE APPARENT INCREASE IN SENSITIVITY?

That is a really good question and I guess there is no one simple answer. The prevalence of both CD and NCGS has been steadily increasing over the last 30 years. It is most likely to be for a number of reasons that there has been a steady increase in the number of people that are being diagnosed with CD or NCGS.

One reason could be the increased awareness in practitioners and the general public which has led to more screening and therefore more frequent diagnosis. Or the change to more sensitive testing, or even that the testing is more widely available. You can now have tests not only ordered by your doctor but also by a variety of health practitioners and I have even seen one type of preliminary screening done in some pharmacies.

Another thing I do find from talking to patients with tummy issues, whether it be wheat/gluten or even dairy causing their reactions. Is that they react very strongly in Australia but when on an overseas holiday in Europe they can tolerate these two food groups. There are some that think it is simply a matter of stress or more to the point, that we are relaxed on our holidays. Stress weakens our digestive system and makes us less capable of efficient digestion. Stress also increases the inflammatory response and more inflammation = more pain.

Something else that has changed in the last 30 years is the way we process grains. There have been so many changes that it would be hard to pinpoint the one culprit. We have been using un-germinated grains and not giving the grain time to ferment. Both of these processes would normally help to breakdown and digest the gluten protein, which makes it far easier for our tummies to digest.

The way bread is made in Australia these days has also changed immensely. My Mum still remembers when my Babcia (Grandma) made bread in Poland, it sat in a cool place to ferment and process for 7 days before baking. This time that was given to proving and fermentation helped develop the bread, breakdown the gluten protein and also increase the beneficial bacteria. These days, bread is no longer made like this, apart from bread that is made by artisan bakers. In Europe they still stick to these traditional methods, which would help to explain why some of my patients can eat a baguette in France without suffering the consequences they would in Australia. (This does not include patients with CD)

In the last 30 years we have also been adding a more refined version of gluten to breads. This means that not only is the content of gluten higher, but it is also more processed. This processed version of gluten or 'vital gluten' as it is known, is much more damaging to our digestive lining as it is stripped of the naturally protective and anti-inflammatory chemicals.

Compared to the old/traditional wheat grains like spelt, the hybridised wheat we use today has something called wheat germ agglutinins. These are very high in hybridised wheat as it is what makes it more resistant to pests. Wheat germ agglutinins are toxic to mould, fungi and insects, so you can see how this would help protect the plant. This leads to higher yield and profits. The affect that wheat germ agglutinins have on us, is to cause inflammation and a weakening of the small intestine lining. This means the good bacteria and food particles can now interact with our immune system to a greater degree and leads to sensitivities and more symptoms with wheat ingestion.

Another big change in the last 15 years is the use of chemical herbicides like glyphosate, just prior to harvesting of grains like wheat. Just like it kills weeds, it is now thought that it has the capacity to attack our healthy gut flora. Healthy gut flora help to protect us by keeping our immune system in balance, processing of foods and many other roles. Glyphosate also decreases our ability to absorb nutrients and affects chemical pathways in our body that are known to influence the development of conditions including CD.

As you can see there have been so many changes to the processing of wheat and also in food manufacturing that they probably all contribute to the increase of gluten sensitivities. And we can't all just move to Europe or be on a holiday forever, unless maybe, we win the lotto. Although none of this would help those with CD.

Chapter 3

WHAT ACTUALLY HAPPENS IN COELIAC DISEASE?

IMPORTANCE OF A STRICT GLUTEN FREE EATING PLAN

Although symptoms can vary considerably in CD, everybody with the condition is at risk of complications if they do not adhere strictly to treatment with a GF diet. There is no correlation between symptoms and bowel damage, so even if you are asymptomatic (you have no obvious symptoms), damage to the small bowel can still occur if gluten is ingested. This means everybody with CD, irrespective of the severity of their symptoms, needs to adhere strictly to a GF diet.

WHAT HAPPENS TO THE GUT LINING?

In CD there is inflammation and damage to the lining of the small intestine which is covered in finger-like projections that are called villi. The villi of the gut lining increase the surface area, which increases the area that is available to help with digestion and absorption of nutrients from the food we eat. When someone with CD consumes anything containing gluten there is a reaction which causes the flattening out of the villi, this is called "villous atrophy". This inflammation and flattening can lead to nutrient deficiencies and also causes immune and inflammation reactions in other organs leading to further complications. The flattening of the villi can be happening even when there are no symptoms.

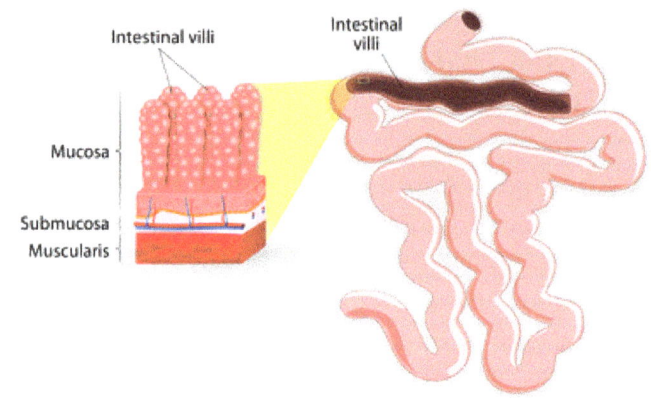

Villi (small finger like projections) line the inside of the small intestine and increase the surface area for absorption and digestion to take place.

WHAT ACTUALLY HAPPENS IN COELIAC DISEASE?

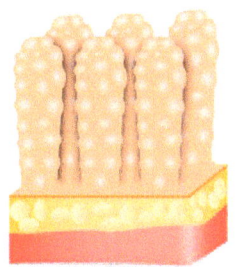

Healthy Villi   Damaged Villi as they can
                     appear in Coeliac disease

Illustration of what healthy villi look like as compared to damaged villi in CD. As you can see they are much smaller and inflamed. This damage hugely affects the small intestines ability to do its job of absorbing food due to the decreased surface area.

Chapter 4

WHAT IF YOUR SYMPTOMS CONTINUE?

If you are continuing to have symptoms even after commencing a GF diet, there are a few things to take into consideration. The first thing is that it can take 12-24 months for your tummy to be restored to full health. We can speed up or at least help this process of healing along by feeding your digestive system the right nutrients to help support healing. While you are healing you may react to lactose or other foods, as your digestive capacity is lower.

It could also be that gluten is sneaking its way into your diet unknowingly. Keeping a comprehensive diet diary of all the foods, drinks, medications and supplements you are ingesting and the symptoms you are experiencing, is a great place to start. Going over this diary with a dietician or health professional specialising in CD, could just make something click or reveal itself.

I know I have had a case of a patient with some symptoms starting, even though they thought they were adhering to a GF diet 100% of the time.

It was when I was reviewing their supplements, that I noticed one of them, actually stated it contained gluten. Even though most medications and supplements these days are made GF, you still need to be vigilant and check every label. I would not have picked this up if he had not actually brought in all the bottles with him.

COULD IT BE CROSS-REACTIVITY?

Some people with CD and NCGS can find that the removal of gluten from the diet does not lead to a complete reversal in symptoms and this can be due to a number of factors. The gut can be severely damaged between the time that the disease starts and when it gets diagnosed. Scientists have noted that it can sometimes take years for complete healing of the lining of the small intestine.

CD can reduce the amount of digestive enzymes secreted as the gut lining is damaged and this can lead to the reduced ability to break down other foods properly, at least until the gut function returns to normal capacity.

If this occurs, then attention should be given to foods that cause cross-reactivity which include yeast, corn, millet, rice and dairy. Please note there is no need to just avoid all these foods without investigation, otherwise it would lead to a very limited diet as corn and rice do usually become a common substitute in GF diets.

ARE FODMAPs AN ISSUE?

FODMAP stands for 'fermentable oligosaccharides,

disaccharides, monosaccharides and polyols'. You can find lots about them online, in books and through many health professionals including Dr.Sue Shepherd who developed the diet. In susceptible individuals the ingestion of foods high in FODMAPs can create a variety of symptoms including diarrhoea, gas and bloating.

This happens because the sugars are not well digested and absorbed, so they spend longer in the digestive tract. Once they are in the large bowel, they draw more water in causing the bloating and diarrhoea. Our normal healthy bacteria also ferment the sugars causing increased bloating, cramping and gas.

The main FODMAPs are:

- Oligosaccharides, such as fructans/fructo-oligosaccharides (found in grains and vegetables) and galactans/galacto-oligosaccharides (found in legumes)
- Disaccharides, such as lactose (found in milk)
- Monosaccharides, such as fructose (found in fruit)
- Polyols, such as sorbitol (found in sweetened products)

To determine if FODMAPs might be contributing to your symptoms, the most effective strategy is to eliminate all FODMAP-containing foods and observe your symptoms. Following the elimination of all FODMAPs, the next step is to complete a systematic rechallenge one-by-one of each FODMAP to help determine the tolerable doses and types of FODMAPs for you. This should be done with the guidance of a health practitioner who understands FODMAPs and can include a dietician or naturopath.

IS SMALL INTESTINE BACTERIAL OVERGROWTH TO BLAME?

Small intestine bacterial overgrowth (SIBO) is a condition where bacteria that may be healthy in other areas of the body, overgrows in the wrong location, in the small intestine. This can lead to a huge variety of symptoms, which do overlap with IBS and other digestive conditions. SIBO can actually be the cause of your IBS symptoms, and there are studies that show it is pres-ent in up to 84% of cases. It also appears to be common in those with Crohn's disease and Diabetes. Symptoms can include constipation, diarrhoea or a mixture of both, cramping, wind, bloating, reflux, skin rashes and iron and B12 deficiencies. You can see how the symptoms do overlap with CD.

It is so important to be properly tested, to see if you are positive and then begin the very specific and effective treatment. Treatment is very complex and needs to be prescribed and monitored by a healthcare practitioner that specialises in SIBO treatment. It involves anti-microbial treatment, digestive repair, nutrient restoration and a very specialised diet.

Not all testing for SIBO is created equal and it is important that you are guided through all the steps. You need to find a practitioner who specialises in treating SIBO, like me. Then you know you are going to get the right testing, effective treatment and invaluable support. You can find more information at www.sibotest.com

IS IT ALSO IRRITABLE BOWEL SYNDROME?

IBS is a syndrome, not a disease. This means it is a collection of symptoms and a doctor will usually conclude you have it, once all other diseases related to you symptoms are ruled out. In other words it is a diagnosis of exclusion. It is a collection of gut symptoms with the main ones being abdominal pain and constipation and/or diarrhoea. Additional symptoms can vary hugely from person to person, but include bloating, cramping, excess wind, sensitivity to foods and reflux.

You may also have been told, there is nothing that can be done to improve the condition apart from taking medications to ease the symptoms. However there are health professionals, including naturopaths like me that can help to relieve your IBS symptoms.

OTHER DIGESTIVE AUTOIMMUNE CONDITIONS

Inflammatory bowel disease (IBD) is a non-specific, chronic inflammatory disease of the digestive system. Both Crohn's disease and Ulcerative Colitis are types of IBD which involve chronic inflammation of the gut lining, both diseases effect different areas of the bowel and different layers. They often present with a pattern of relapses, followed by symptom free periods. Nutritional deficiencies due to malabsorption are common, just like in CD. The other digestive symptoms and fatigue are also shared with CD and it is possible to have both IBD and CD. The IBD conditions are conclusively diagnosed through colonoscopies and tissue samples being taken. There is also a new test called Calprotectin which is a stool sample, so less invasive. This is a possible first step to see if you have high levels of this inflammatory marker, which is common in IBD and gut infections, as it is an indicator of tissue damage. This test alone does not give a diagnosis. You can have this test done with a gastroenterologist or even a naturopath who deals with gut issues and offers laboratory testing.

Chapter 5

WHY A GLUTEN FREE DIET MAY NOT BE ENOUGH

When the small intestine is in an acute state of inflammation and is damaged as described previously, there are many functions that are affected. The gut lining has many jobs to do, it is considered the body's largest immune organ and is the host's greatest source of contact with the environment. It is estimated that about 80% of our body's immune defence cells live in this tissue. The gut lining provides a barrier, digestive enzymes to assist breakdown of food and is how the nutrients from what we eat enter our blood stream. Your digestive system is very, very busy! Below is a pictorial version of all the areas we need to consider in digestive health. One or multiple areas can be affected at the one time.

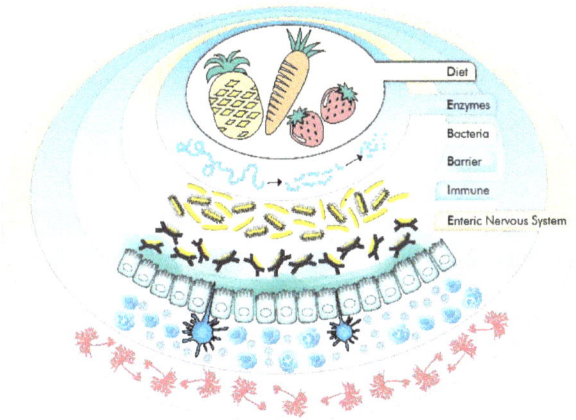

Diagram provided by Metagenics PTY.LTD.

THE BARRIER

Our digestive system has many linings, our oesophagus, stomach lining, small intestine and large intestine. They are all made of tissue called mucous membrane. All these linings or barriers protect the rest of our body from what happens in these organs and also performs many functions. We wouldn't want stomach acid spilling into the rest of our body, so in this case it protects us from the very corrosive acids. The stomach lining also produces digestive enzymes to assist with breaking down our food. We want our barriers to be strong, tight and intact so they can function as intended, allowing the passage of nutrients and water, whilst preventing or limiting the movement of pathogens, toxins or allergens across the lining. When someone is diagnosed with CD their gut is very porous and leaky, making it easier for gluten and other allergens to affect the immune system. Intestinal permeability or a "leaky gut" has been linked to many disorders including CD, IBD, eczema, asthma, other allergies, weight gain and rheumatoid arthritis.

One of the aims of treatment in CD is to repair this lining. Avoiding gluten will stop further damage and give the gut the time and opportunity to heal and repair. Simply avoiding gluten can mean that it can be years before the lining of the gut is healed and some studies have shown that the mucosal gut lining has not normalised even after five years.

There are many factors that drive the breakdown of the tight junctions between the cells in our gut lining. In every person I see in clinic it is important to start healing the gut and identify and address the factors that may be driving the inflammation and breakdown of the gut lining. There is no point continually trying to heal the lining if you are going to be constantly exposing it to what is irritating it. This is another reason that someone with CD or NCGS should be very strict with their diet.

The other factors that need to be considered in the healing of barriers:

Antibiotics	Radiation and chemotherapy
Trauma or stress	Other food allergies
Excess alcohol	Imbalance in gut flora

Viral and bacterial gastroenteritis	Oral contraceptive pill
Non-steroidal anti-inflammatory drugs	

(This information does not mean you should abruptly cease any medications, you must always consult your general practitioner)

Naturopathy has a whole dispensary of nutrients and herbs available to heal, repair and decrease inflammation of the digestive system. This helps to support and speed up healing and gives symptomatic relief quite quickly.

THE DIGESTIVE ENZYMES

Digestive enzymes are produced in the small intestine lining but there are also chemicals produced here that orchestrate the release of pancreatic digestive enzymes. Digestive enzymes make sure we are breaking down our food into small enough particles, so that they can be absorbed across the gut lining. If the correct breakdown does not occur and you have a " leaky" gut lining, larger that appropriate particles are absorbed and can create more immune reactions and it can also cause more pain and discomfort in your tummy.

It has been shown that even after the removal of gluten from the diet someone with CD has a reduced function of the secretory cells. In particular the cells that secrete lactase (which breaks down lactose from dairy products) seem to be under functioning. It is important to consider supporting digestive enzyme secretion, so that you do not get cross-reactivity to other foods while the tummy is still healing.

Naturopathy has supplements that can replace your digestive enzymes while your body is healing and struggling to produce the right amount of these enzymes. As your body recovers it is then worth supporting and stimulating your body's own ability to produce these digestive enzymes itself. The right volume of each of the digestive enzymes is essential for proper digestion and absorption of minerals taken from the foods we eat. We need to be able to break down the protein, fats and carbohydrates that we ingest into small enough particles so that they can be absorbed correctly. If incomplete digestion occurs we can experience many symptoms including gas, bloating, diarrhoea, pain and it also puts more strain on the immune system.

THE DIET

To be on a GF diet and to do it well and be happy and healthy can be difficult. Gluten can be hidden in almost all processed foods. It is not as simple as avoiding the obvious sources like bread, pasta and baked goods. Similarly, having one appointment with a dietician or your specialist is not enough. To be GF, happy and healthy you need lots of support from family and friends. Also do lots of reading and educate yourself on the subject as much as you can. This will make it much easier and enjoyable to be strictly GF.

Research has shown that around 50-80% of patients with CD are not 100% compliant on their GF diet. This can include the consumption of non-GF drinks like beer.

Some individuals may still consume it from time to time as they miss it (totally understandable). They do not realise the damage it is really doing, their symptoms may not be too bad with small amounts or they just may not truly understand the significant damage it does.

With a damaged gut lining and decreased digestion and absorption it is easy to see why people with CD can become deficient in a range of vitamins and minerals. The most common nutrient deficiencies are iron, B12 and folic acid as these are largely absorbed in the exact area that is damaged during a CD flare up.

Other nutrients that may also be low are:

Vitamin D, Vitamin K, Vitamin B6, Zinc, Selenium and Copper

Always seek professional advice before taking high doses of nutrients, especially if you are currently taking other medications.

BACTERIA

There is more and more evidence that the balance of bacteria in the gut lining is disrupted in both CD and NCGS. It is thought to be part of the condition but also to worsen the symptoms of these conditions. Correcting this issue will not cure the person but it can definitely help to improve symptoms, improve the function of the digestive system and may even provide some protection against other autoimmune conditions.

There have been studies done on patients with CD that

have been on a strict GF diet but still have gut symptoms present like diarrhoea, gas, bloating and abdominal pain. In one study of 15 people, 10 tested positive to SIBO (small intestinal bacteria overgrowth), and 2 had parasitic infections. This demonstrates that the GF diet alone could not correct all the gut symptoms that were occurring in these patients. Without addressing the bacteria imbalance then it will continue to affect the health of the gut lining and possibly lead to more complications.

Chapter 6

ASSOCIATED MEDICAL CONDITIONS

There are a range of diseases that are associated with the presence of CD and you need to know what they are. So that you can be aware of the symptoms and so you can be screened for these conditions too. There are a number of reasons that these associations are present.

CD has a genetic predisposition, which means you inherit the genes from your parents that can make you more susceptible to developing CD if certain triggers occur in your life. These genes are also associated with other autoimmune conditions. The two most common conditions that CD is associated with are Autoimmune Thyroid Disease and Type I Diabetes. Due to this genetic link you can find a variety of immune related conditions in one family, even if everyone does not have CD they may have any number of other autoimmune diseases.

So if an immediate family member has an autoimmune condition or someone else in your family has CD it is worth screening everyone for CD. There are studies now showing the longer CD is left untreated, the more likely the person is to develop other related autoimmune conditions. As we know not everyone with CD has clear and obvious symptoms, it is important to have the testing done.

Another complication of untreated CD as mentioned previously, is that it impairs your absorption of nutrients. This means that no matter how healthy your diet is, due to the inflammation going on in the small intestine, not a lot of nutrients may be making it into your blood stream to be used by the rest of your body. Other organs can be affected by this same inflammation that is occurring in the gut and cause complications like osteoporosis, infertility, anaemia and liver disease.

The following conditions tend to occur at higher rates in people with CD, it can be due to the genetic, immune, inflammatory or malabsorption component. This list is classified into the different body systems and was taken from information produced by Coeliac Australia.

Endocrine/Hormonal system

Autoimmune thyroid disease, type I diabetes, Addison's disease (insufficient adrenal hormones), Sjogren's syndrome (dry mouth & eyes), Amenorrhoea (absence of periods)

Joints

Rheumatoid arthritis, polyarthritis, lupus (body attacks

healthy tissue & joints), sarcoidosis (inflamed nodules in lungs).

Blood

Anaemia, chronic low platelets.

Gastrointestinal

Lactose intolerance, pernicious anaemia (inability to absorb B12), pancreatic insufficiency (inability to properly digest food), microscopic diarrhoea (watery diarrhoea), gastrointestinal cancers.

Bone

Premature osteopaenia (low bone density), osteoporosis, rickets or osteomalacia (caused by low vitamin D).

Liver

Abnormal liver function tests, autoimmune hepatitis, blocked bile ducts, scarring of bile ducts.

Nervous system

Multiple sclerosis, epilepsy, depression, neuropathy (breakdown of nervous tissue).

Skin and mouth

Dermatitis herpetiformis, alopecia, dental enamel defects, mouth ulcers.

Reproductive system

Infertility, recurrent miscarriage.

Chapter 7

IMPROVING YOUR DIGESTIVE HEALTH AND WHAT TO DO DURING ACUTE ATTACKS

WHAT YOU CAN DO TO IMPROVE YOUR DIGESTIVE HEALTH

Dietary tips

- Enjoy liberal amounts of fruits and vegetables for nutrient, prebiotic and fibre effects.

- Eat good quality protein to improve barrier function.

- Enjoy food such as bitter greens (rocket, endive) and sour fruits to stimulate digestion.

- Enjoy fermented foods like sauerkraut for probiotic effects.

- Avoid or minimise potential dietary irritants such as preservatives, smoked and charred foods, coffee and alcohol.

- Don't drink ice cold drinks, as they can irritate a sensitive tummy.

- Soups and slightly cooked warm foods are more supportive of digestion, than raw and uncooked foods. This may be especially important when you are newly diagnosed or suffering with a lot of digestive symptoms, as your gut is most likely inflamed and under-functioning.

- Avoid excessively spicy, greasy or deep-fried foods.

- Reduce dairy products.

- Avoid processed and overcooked foods. Make sure to reheat food correctly, if not hot enough you could be ingesting bacteria that can cause further irritation.

- Monitor individual foods and adjust diet accordingly. It is much easier to notice the effects certain foods have on you after completing a cleanse and repair program. Always do this with the guidance of a health professional.

Lifestyle tips – it's not just what you eat, but how you eat

- Sit down & relax when you are eating.

- Avoid eating when stressed, your blood is taken away from the stomach meaning you will not breakdown your food as well and this can cause many symptoms.

- Eat mindfully –when eating, just eat. Try to avoid

watching TV, working or reading. Concentrate on the flavour and textures, this will stimulate your digestion.

- Eat with family and friends whenever possible as it is so much more enjoyable.

- Chew your food thoroughly, this is the very beginning of digestion.

- Avoid excessive fluid consumption with meals.

- Get involved in the food preparation and cook with love.

- Eat until you are about 80% full, this means you are eating until you are no longer hungry but not full.

- Eating slowly and mindfully is very important for the above tip, as it takes at least 12 minutes from when you start eating, for your brain to register that you are full. So if you eat quickly then you can easily overeat.

WHAT TO DO WHEN YOU GET GLUTEN'ED'

From time to time, no matter how vigilant you are with your diet and avoiding gluten from all sources, you will be exposed to some. In some individuals even small amounts of gluten will cause pain, discomfort nausea and/or vomiting. These types of symptoms can last hours to days and are accompanied by damage to your intestinal lining. Even if you do not experience painful symptoms, you will have done damage to your intestinal lining if you have CD. Your immune system reacts every time it is exposed to gluten, not only to large amounts.

If you have NCGS then you may have very unpleasant symptoms but they will not be accompanied by the cellular damage that is present in CD. Even taking this into consideration, you will have inflammation and the advice during and following acute attacks would be the same.

Naturopathy can be of great value during these times as it can help to alleviate symptoms. Generally there are no medications that are recommended during this time, you are told to just wait it out.

The following tips may help:

- Avoiding all gluten and dairy (dairy only during the initial acute attack).
- Eating foods that are easy to digest and are gentle on the stomach and intestines as you will have compromised digestion at this time. Soups and plenty of vegetables are a great idea.
- Eating slowly and chewing thoroughly will be especially important, so that you help your body with digestion.
- Avoiding fatty, processed, sugary foods and alcohol is important as they cause more inflammation and can therefore slow healing and worsen symptoms.
- Choosing chicken and fish over red meat, like a heavy steak or sausages, is a good idea as they are easier to process. Fish is also anti-inflammatory.
- Strictly avoiding any other foods that you know do not agree with you is especially important at this time.

- Dealing with stress and enjoying lots of relaxation is important as stress can have a very negative effect on gut health.

- If you are experiencing cramping pain then a wheat bag or hot pack, can help to ease the pain, as can a warm bath with Epsom salts.

- Supporting digestion with the use of lemon juice or apple cider vinegar, diluted in water before meals, will help to stimulate your digestion.

Reducing intestinal permeability, supporting digestion, restoring appropriate bacterial balance and controlling tissue damage at this time can all be addressed with natural supplements. A specific plan can be drawn up for someone by me after consultation and discussion of their condition and common symptoms. Natural supplements can speed up the healing process and quickly reduce any digestive symptoms, getting you back to enjoying life and food again as soon as possible.

If you are gluten sensitive (but do not have Coeliac disease), there are some supplements available to help you break down gluten better so that it may cause less symptoms if you know you are going to ingest gluten. This is not recommended in CD as you really do need to be 100% strict with your diet.

Chapter 8

THE HEART OF THE HOME – THE KITCHEN

In our household, which only included my husband and I at the time he was first diagnosed with CD, we found it easiest to take everything out of the pantry and fridge. We then put aside all the gluten-containing foods to give to family and friends, returned all the safe foods to the fridge and started looking at what we could replace with GF alternatives. I did keep the normal flours for a while, as I love baking and thought I would use them when making things for friends parties etc. But they ended up going off, I chucked them out and never replaced them. While we had everything out of the fridge and pantry, we gave it all a good scrub to remove any crumbs and residues. Another thing we got rid of was the spreads, as they may contain hidden crumbs, from double dipping. The toaster is one item you may choose to replace if the whole household is going GF or you could have two of them. I have been told by some dieticians that it is fine to use the same one. They do collect a lot of crumbs, so cleaning out often will be necessary and it really is what you feel comfortable with.

There are benefits to the whole household going GF and there are benefits to not doing this. It really is a very individual case and depends on who makes up your family and what is best for each member. When it was just my husband and I, we had everything GF, except for my bread (mainly due to cost). But once our daughter started eating solids, we did start including some non-GF staples such as crackers and bread, but this is very easy to keep separate. We both wanted her to be exposed to gluten while her digestive system is maturing. We did this so that she does not develop sensitivity or intolerance from never having had it. However, for all the meals I prepare and bake I do so GF.

If you have numerous GF children in your household, you may choose to colour code items, red for not safe and green for safe. Or you could even just have a container or two filled with GF foods with the child's name or some stickers on it. This way they know anything in these containers is safe and they don't necessarily need to ask you every time. There are so many ways of dealing with the fridge and pantry, you just need to find a system or rules that best fit in with your family. Even though my daughter is too young to read and my husband can read labels, we still have a large box with non-GF snacks for her and a GF box for him. Everything else in our fridge and pantry is GF.

If the whole family is not going GF, everyone will need to be mindful of cross contamination. Wiping down surfaces, chopping boards is very important. As well as not using the same utensils to stir a GF dish and a non-GF dish. Once washed though all cutlery, glassware, utensils and plates and bowls are safe to use with any foods. When using a spread like butter, nut spreads, jam and honey no double dipping should be done, so do use separate knives. I always prepare the GF toast first, then I can use that knife on my daughter's bread. You will develop your own systems and habits.

When storing foods in the fridge or freezer especially, it can be useful to label whether it is GF or not, so there is no confusion later on. As I rarely cook with gluten containing ingredients, I only label them as NOT GF when needed. This more often happens when someone gives me food for our daughter to take home.

In the beginning it is normal to be apprehensive about changing your cooking and recipes. But you do develop an understanding of how the GF flours and ingredients work and you will find amazing alternatives and get so good at it, that people may not be able to tell it's GF. I remember in the beginning, I would be half way through cooking dinner and have this sudden panic, that I used an ingredient with gluten in it. Or that I forgot to check all the labels. I would race to the pantry or fridge and speedily read the label to make sure I wasn't going to "poison" my husband. If this happens to you, don't worry you are normal (or at least I like to think it's normal, because I did it so often) and it will stop. You will become a pro at knowing what's safe straight away. But it is still worth checking labels from time to time and I still do this, as things with manufacturers can change.

Chapter 9

BRINGING HAPPY BACK

Being diagnosed with any lifelong condition means some changes for the person, whether it is dietary, lifestyle or adjusting to taking some medication or supplements. For someone newly diagnosed with CD it can include all of these changes. Some people find these changes harder than others, it depends on so many factors including their age, previous symptoms, how long they have had symptoms for, their family situation, knowledge of food and its ingredients and their current diet. At first there could be shock and grief, "Why me?", "But I have always eaten wheat and been fine" or "Is it forever?" On the other hand some people that have been suffering with severe symptoms for a lifetime may have a feeling of relief, " finally an answer", "now it all makes sence".

No matter what your initial reaction is, there are some major and lifelong changes that need to be made and they really do involve every aspect of your life, oh and it all needs to happen immediately. No slow weening off the gluten that is now seen by your body as an evil enemy. Whether you are eating at home, socialising over a meal or packing your food for school or work, your new GF diet needs to be taken into consideration. There is a lot to learn and adjust to and quick smart.

Our first stop after the appointment with the dietician was FREE on Unley Road. This is a store that only stock GF products. We thought our first stop should be a GF haven. It felt very safe to go there, buy up big and know we wouldn't be making any mistakes. After our purchases we sat down there had a coffee and drowned our sorrows over a car-amel GF cupcake (not the most naturopathic snack or that great for stress, but I am human too).Even as a naturopath it was a tad overwhelming for me at first. I had only done GF for three months at a time before, not for life.

There has been a lot of purchasing, trying and sometimes discarding of food that we found inedible. Now after 3.5 years of living GF, we have our favourites and know where to get them from and how to adapt our recipes. We know what questions to ask before my husband eats anything, at friends places or at restaurants, as we know where the sneaky little gluten may be hiding. We pretty much have a handle on all aspects of GF eating, not that I am saying it's easy all the time.

This is where I want to talk about the part that makes it a little hard sometimes and I guess would not really be discussed at your dietician's appointment. No matter how much you know and how well you can stick to the GF diet. I think it is very important to not overlook one aspect. It is the emotional toll that it can have on the person with CD and even on their family to a certain extent. Stress and depression can have a huge affect on how well you deal with the condition, your quality of life and preventing any other complications, as we now know stress can trigger many conditions.

It can take many years to get over a shock and being diagnosed with a chronic condition is definitely a shock. Having CD does change many aspects of your life, like the ease of eating out, the cost of food, travelling, confidence, self love and self esteem. Also the amount of pleasure that you derive from eating and sharing a meal with others can change. Sometimes it can feel like you are left out of certain situations, especially when you do not feel comfortable asking about GF options. You may feel that everything you love and enjoy has been taken away from you, I know that my husband still feels like this from time to time. All these feelings are normal, but if they start taking over or becoming overwhelming it is something you need to talk to family, friends or even a professional about.

Many people do not understand the seriousness of this condition and just how important it is to remain 100% GF. Even if you have NCGS, it can be so important for you to be strict but others may not understand. You need to remember you are not being fussy or trying to cause a problem, this is what you must do to remain healthy. My husband prefers if I am the one ordering and asking the questions on his behalf, then he does not need to be the one taking the occasional rudeness or bluntness of staff. I find it easier than him to explain how serious it is that the food be GF and I always make sure that people I am talking to actually know and understand what I mean. We never take a risk if it seems like they may not completely understand what gluten is found in, we simply move onto another restaurant. Like one night while travelling interstate, we called a restaurant and I start to ask my usual questions, they respond with "yes our food is GF", followed a few minutes later by "What is gluten?". As you can imagine, I thanked them and moved on. Now we just laugh about these situations.

It is getting better and easier to go out and eat but you still need to be very vigilant. You may find it easier if someone does the questioning for you too. I think it's always easier if someone asks on your behalf, although obviously this is not always possible.

Talking about how you feel to others, what is hard, easy and how far you have come is important.

Telling all your family, friends and work colleagues about your condition is very important, so that they understand the needs you might have at get togethers and functions. We always offer to bring a plate and that way we know that there will be at least one thing for my husband to eat. It does not make you feel great if you go to a party and can't touch any of the food, it's all part of socialising.

Anyone who loves beer needs to tell everyone that they can no longer drink it (apart from the GF varieties of course). That way when you get to the pub, you don't have to start explaining why you can't take part in the rounds or do not feel weird about asking for a wine or cider instead. I have seen this in my husband's case as he loves beer, especially craft, German and Polish beers.

Trying new recipes and learning to adjust them can make you feel more in control and happy. To know that you can still enjoy your favourite meal, even if some of them are only at home. Being involved in the food preparation can help, especially for children. They are usually more willing to try new meals, when they are part of the process.

I believe reading books, magazines and even blogs on the subject can make you feel a part of a community who completely understands what you are going through. It can help to give you new ideas or suggestions. It can stop you feeling like you are on your own, or you are the only one who has multiple conditions.

By asking questions when you are out and explaining that you have CD, I have found myself having many conversations with new people about their experiences or the experiences of someone they know. It's amazing how many people are out there, who can actually help you by offering some info or a tip about a new product or place to eat.

Herbal and nutritional supplements can offer you support for the emotional aspect. There are herbs that can improve your resilience to stress and help you cope with some of the emotions.

Feelings of stress and depression can also be due to

nutritional deficiencies, so I believe you should always have full blood tests done to screen for vitamin and mineral deficiencies, as this is very common at the time of diagnosis. For example simply being iron deficient can produce symptoms of anxiety. If you know what you are deficient in, you can take high quality, easily digested and absorbed supplements to correct the deficiencies as soon as possible. It is very important especially with all the damage in the gut in the initial stages, that you use supplements that are easily absorbed.

Things you might like to try

- Meditation

- Hypnotherapy

Joining communities online including following people on Instagram – this can stop you feeling alone and give you tons of recipes and inspiration to continue with your own journey

Read gluten free blogs and books – for the above reasons

If you have never really cooked much, just try. It definitely makes you happy to create yummy gluten free food. Or even enrol in some cooking classes if you need some more pointers.

Treat yourself to some delish raw treats, there are so many cafes that stock them these days. They always make me happy. (Raw treats are gluten, dairy and added sugar free desserts, they can be true master pieces these days.)

Subscribing to magazines like *Australian Gluten Free*

Life or *Yum* can provide lots of information, recipes and suggestions of making life better. It also makes you feel like part of a community.

Chapter 10

GLUTEN FREE DIET IN CHILDREN AND TEENS

Children

If it is your child who is diagnosed with CD or intolerance, then that brings a whole new set of emotions as the parent. You may feel responsible, like you didn't do enough (especially if the diagnosis was a long and slow process), scared for them, protective and it will add a lot of stress to your daily life for a while. All your emotions are normal, but it is really important not to blame yourselves.

Depending on their age, they will have tried a different variety of gluten containing foods. In some ways though kids are far more resilient, then us 'tough' adults and they may not grieve in the same way for the foods. Especially if you learn to make pretty good substitutes for their favourites. Nicole Hun writes a blog and books on making all your favourite foods GF. You can find her on 'Gluten Free on a Shoestring'.

Do the most important things now, like cleaning out the pantry and informing their daycare, kindy or school of the changes. It depends on their age how much and how you to choose to explain this to them. I believe just stick to the most important things they need to know and don't go into all the information about labels and complications of CD. This will be something you slowly discuss as they get older. Kids are more likely to have accidental ingestions of gluten containing foods and they will quickly be able to see how sick it makes them. This will be especially true as the gut heals and the sensitivity and reactions increase due to the immune system recovering and in a way being stronger.

If you have numerous children in your household, you may choose to colour code items, red for not safe and green for safe. Or you could even just have a container or two filled with GF foods with the child's name or some stickers on it. This way they know anything in these containers is safe and they don't necessarily need to ask you every time. There are so many ways of dealing with the fridge and pantry, you just need to find a system or rules that best fit in with your family. Even though my daughter is too young to read and my husband can read labels, we stick have a large box with non-GF snacks for her and a GF box for him. Everything else in our fridge and pantry is GF.

Teenagers

Teenagers, teenagers....what can we say, they can be a tricky bunch at the best of times. This is probably one of the harder times to be 100% GF, as there is such a strong social aspect in their life. Also peer pressure and the way you appear to others is so important. Who wants to ask their friend to read a label before they consume the chips or chocolate that are being shared around. My husband would even hate to do that. Not many of us want to be the centre of attention in that situation.

It probably really depends on how long they have been doing the GF diet for, what their reactions are like when they do ingest gluten and the friends they have around them. They may want to rebel against it, or show they can have control of their bodies. This will be a bigger problem if your child has a more silent type of CD or intolerance, as you won't necessarily have clear cut symptoms. Early discussions and knowledge about the damage gluten can do and the importance of a GF diet, will make it much easier to handle in teenage years.

Chapter 11

YOUR EVERYDAY LIVING RESOURCE

FOODS CONTAINING GLUTEN

Wheat, triticale, rye, barley and oats must always be avoided. Do not consume any of these products unless clearly and specifically labelled as a GF alternative. For example you can now buy GF breadcrumbs or GF oats. Do not use food labelled as low gluten foods, without reading the ingredients label.

Wheat and triticale – found in

- All normal breads, rolls and wraps, even spelt, wholemeal and multigrain
- Wheat starch
- Wheat & multigrain flour, bran & wheat germ
- Wheat based cereals & mueslis
- Biscuits, infant rusks, cakes, pasta, crackers, noodles
- Semolina

- Crumbed or coated foods, like fish, meats and even many hot chips these days
- Breadcrumbs and batters
- Some sausages and processed meats
- Gravy , some sauces, salad dressings
- Some baking powders & cornflours
- Starches & thickeners derived from wheat
- Wafers, waffles, pancakes, doughnuts, croissants, pastries
- Coffee substitutes like Caro and some hot chocolates
- Triticale flour, cereals, some grains like cous cous
- Icing sugar mixtures
- Vegemite
- Some varieties of chocolate, any that have wafers & biscuit pieces
- Some ice-creams

Rye-found in

- Rye breads, crisp breads eg. Rye vita & pumpernickel breads

Barley-found in

- Barley, pearl barley, barley flour
- Barley bread & biscuits

- Soups containing barley or pearl barley
- Malt, malted cereals, malt extract
- Malted milks & chocolate flavoured drinks like Milo & ovaltine
- Barley drinks & lollies
- Beer
- Cereal coffee alternatives like caro
- Some chocolates like Lindt balls & maltesers

Oats – Found in

- Oats, porridge, muesli & muesli bars
- Oat cakes & Anzac biscuits
- Oat bran & oat flour
- Haggis
- Oat containing cereals
- Sough dough breads (even if made with gluten free flour be aware that some starter cultures for sough dough bread contain oats)

INGREDIENTS CONTAINING GLUTEN

Reading food labels

This is a very useful and important skill when following a strict GF diet. Doing it well means not eliminating unnecessary foods or accidentally ingesting gluten. It is handy while shopping in the supermarket, eating at someone's house or eating out at a restaurant. Not all foods in the supermarket that are GF are marked across the front or even found in the GF isle. On so many occasions while eating out or eating at a friend's I have checked a label of a product they have used to double check. It not only means not consuming gluten but means that you do not have to miss out on eating something or not at all just because the person preparing or selling the food is not 100% sure it is GF.

The introduction of the new Foods Standards Code in 2002 has made it much easier to read labels and determine if they contain gluten in any way. Even ingredients that are derived from a gluten containing food must be stated on the label. For example if wheat starch is used, it must be labelled as **starch (wheat)** or **wheaten starch** not just **starch**.

If however the starch came from a GF source the manufacturer would not necessarily have to state the ingredient on the label. Most though choose to put it in the ingredient list and when it is from a GF source, they can label it as **starch** or **starch (maize)**.

It is worth noting that if a food contains one of the most common allergens like gluten, egg, dairy, soy, nuts or fish, most manufacturers put this ingredient in **bold lettering**. Making it easier to quickly identify gluten or other allergen foods. However it is not like this 100% of the time, so care should still be taken when reading the label so that you do not miss something.

After the ingredient list there may also be an allergen warning, or a warning stating that the food may contain traces of gluten or other allergens. When it states that it may contain traces of gluten, this is usually because it was manufactured in a factory that is also making gluten containing foods. You will find that these foods are not labelled GF on the front even though they may be.

It is also worth noting that there are some ingredients that even if they are derived from wheat but are so highly processed that there is no trace of gluten left. This means that it is safe to eat, one example is **glucose syrup (wheat)**. It may be **in bold,** state that it is from wheat and even have an allergen statement advising that it contains wheat. But if it was only the glucose syrup from wheat and all other ingredients were GF, it means you could eat it and it would not be on your avoid list.

Food additives

The following food additives are all gluten free, even if made from wheat or other gluten containing grains.

Acidity regulators	Enzymes	Minerals salts
Anti-caking agents	Flavour enhancers	Preservatives
Anti-oxidants	Flavours	Propellants
Artificial sweeteners	Flour treatment agents	Stabilisers
Colour retention agents	Food acids	Vegetable gums
Colours	Glazing agents	
Emulsifiers	Humectants	

All other ingredients made from wheat or gluten containing grains may contain residual amounts of gluten and so must not be consumed.

Compounding ingredients

When a food like a muesli bar is made of many ingredients, all ingredients that make up more than 5% of the finished product must be listed with its individual ingredients too. For example a choc chip muesli bar, would list chocolate chips (cocoa, cocoa butter, sugar). If the chocolate chips made up less than 5% of the bar then it would not have to include the separate ingredients, **unless the chocolate chips were made with a gluten containing grain.** So if it is just listed with 'chocolate chips' then you can assume it is GF.

Processing aids

An example of this is when small chocolates are made, the moulds may be dusted with wheat starch to make them easy to remove. If a processing aid containing gluten is used it must be stated on the label.

'Gluten Free' VS ' Low Gluten'

Foods that are labelled gluten free have been tested and show to contain less that 0.002 grams of gluten per 100grams of food. They will be labelled on the nutritional panel as either 'no detectable gluten' or 'nil' or '0' gluten.

Any foods that are labelled 'low gluten' are not acceptable on a gluten free diet.

Please note that it is worth checking labels of foods regularly, even if they are foods that you have found to be safe. Manufacturers can change the ingredients of their products at any stage, so it is definitely worth quickly scanning the label each time you buy a food that is not specifically labelled as 'Gluten Free'. Once you become a pro at this it is a task that takes a few seconds.

QUICK REFERENCE TO READING FOOD LABELS

GLUTEN FREE INGREDIENTS If written on the label as....	INGREDIENTS TO AVOID If written on the label as....
Cornflour Maize cornflour	Wheaten cornflour
Corn starch Starch Pregel starch Maize starch Potato starch Tapioca starch Modified starch Modified potato starch Modified corn starch	Wheat starch Pregel wheat starch Modified wheat starch
Thickener (modified starch) Thickener (from maize)	Thickener (from wheat)
Yeast Yeast extract	Brewer's yeast Brewer's yeast extract

Rice malt Maltodextrin Maize maltodextrin Soy maltodextrin Dextrin	Malt, malt extract Malt extract (from barley) Wheat maltodextrin Maltodextrin (from wheat) Wheat dextrin
Vinegar	Malt vinegar
Hydrolysed vegetable protein Hydrolysed soy protein Hydrolysed maize protein	Hydrolysed wheat protein
Textured vegetable protein Textured soy protein Textured maize protein	Textured wheat protein
Glucose Glucose syrup Glucose (from wheat) Glucose syrup (from wheat)	
Caramel colour Caramel colour (from wheat) Caramel colour (from maize)	

MEDICATION & SUPPLEMENTS

You must check all your medication and supplements before taking them to make sure they are GF. Wheat is often used as a filler. This includes prescription and over the counter medications, even if your doctor knows you have CD, please check the label or ask the pharmacist to check for you before purchasing.

ALCOHOL

When it comes to alcohol, there is one big no, no...Beer! Unfortunately for anyone who is a beer lover this definitely needs to be avoided. As my husband says nothing tastes like a good beer, especially if you like the darker, heavier ones like the German style beers.

There are GF beers available in Australia, below is a current list, but micro-breweries are coming out with more and more.

Billabong brewing – Australian Pale Ale, Blonde, Ginger, Apple

O'Brien brewing – Premium Lager, Brown Ale, Pale Ale, Natural Light

Schnitzer Brau – Premium Lager, Citrus

You should be able to purchase these from Dan Murphy's.

I have heard more and more, that people think Corona is GF as it is made from corn. Unfortunately this is not true and Corona will even tell you this. Although corn is one of the ingredients it is still brewed with Barley Malt, which contains gluten. It does not matter that you don't notice any symptoms following a few, if you have CD, it is still a no.

All other alcoholic drinks are ok, like wine and spirits, as spirits are distilled. But you need to take care with the mixers. If a drink did contain added gluten, as with food labels it would need to be stated on the label.

TRAVELLING

Flying

Most airlines can provide GF meals, you can contact them or check their website. When making a booking through a travel agent, make them aware of your dietary needs. Also upon check in you can double check that it is noted on your seat that you require GF meals.

After travelling to Europe in 2014 with my husband, we highly recommend that you pack some of your own food and snacks, unless you are happy to go a bit hungry. There was no issue of them knowing he needed the GF meals, but my husband did find some of the meals/snacks were not really edible (although some of us might think that is all plane food). So I can assure you on our return flights we had a GF sandwhich and some snacks.

Travelling overseas

This will obviously always be easier if you are travelling somewhere where English is the main language, as you can easily explain your situation. It does get a bit trickier when travelling somewhere where no or little English is spoken. But definitely doable and so worth it as travelling is such a joy, well for us anyway. With some research and preparation you can definitely make things easier for yourself or a family member. The internet helps so much in this situation.

We travelled to Germany, Poland and Ireland. Ireland was very easy due to being able to speak English and we found they had many GF options marked on the menu when eating out. I thought Germany would be easier than Poland as they speak more English, but Poland was a little easier for us as I can almost speak fluent Polish.

We used these cards that explained my husband has CD and what his dietary restrictions were. I thought this would help us immensely when eating out, as you do so much of that on holidays. I definitely felt more comfortable having them all printed out and ready to go. It did help some of the time, but most of the time it hindered us, as I believe the wait staff got scared and just said "no, nothing here".

We stayed in apartments and it was easier to shop in the supermarket and be able to read the labels and prepare a lot of our own meals. We always took snacks and a sandwhich for the day, just in case we were not able to find somewhere to eat. We had to be prepared due to the type 1 diabetes, when you need to eat , you need to eat quite quickly. Please do not be scared off though, as we did find places to eat and a lot of people were amazingly helpful. Once you find a couple of great places, you just tend to revisit them.

Doing research before leaving is vital. Research where you might find the closest health food stores, or possible shops and restaurants. We found a great health food shop in Berlin and paid them a few visits over our stay.

As I said Poland was easier for the simple fact that I could explain we needed meals without flour, breadcrumbs and sauces and I didn't have to use the translated card that seemed to scare everyone off. Once you know the type of dishes in a country that are safe, you can go from there.

EATING OUT

Parties at home

If you are invited to a party at someone's house, I always advise that you eat a meal before you leave. In our experience this is the best way to avoid being left feeling hungry. If you have eaten then you can easily wait till there is something safe. We always call the host and offer to bring a plate too, so that my husband has something that he knows is 100% safe. Always bring your needs to the attention of the host. Parties are very busy especially for the host, who has a million things on their mind. So even if they had intended to serve lots of GF foods, sometimes they don't make it out of the kitchen. Or possibly the GF foods get mixed in with non GF options.

Parties at function centres

This can be a little trickier, especially if there is no formal invite asking about dietary requirements. It really depends how comfortable you feel discussing your dietary requirements, but I truly believe you need to do this well before the party. Call the host and let them know you will require GF foods, this way the kitchen has plenty of time to prepare. If it is a cocktail party, then when you arrive approach the wait staff and inform them that you are the guest that needs some GF options. It not like it's written across your forehead.

You will probably get a variety of reactions from time to time, I guess it just depends on their knowledge. I find the nicer you ask and the more you can explain, the better your result. If the first staff member you ask isn't sure just ask if they can find out for you or ask someone else.

You just need to get comfortable with discussing your health issue so that people can understand where you are coming from. My husband still hates making a fuss and drawing attention to himself so I find I still do all the talking, but I really don't mind. I do think it is a bit easier if someone else does it for you. Having said all this, still make the effort to have a substantial meal before leaving home or you will end up hungry and it's not as simple as picking up some late night takeaway on the way home.

Another tip is to position yourself closer to the kitchen door, to ensure the GF options do not get eaten up before the tray reaches you.

Restaurants/Cafes

I always advise calling a restaurant before you decide to eat there if you have enough time to plan ahead, unless you have been there recently and know that there are GF options that cater to your tastes. Also just because they say they have GF options, does not mean they will have something substantial or anything that you are happy to pay for. We have called a restaurant, they have said they can do GF so we drive there, only to find out their GF option is a salad with no dressing or meat. So now if we are going somewhere new, I always call to ask if they have GF options and what they actually are or have a quick look at their online menu. That way we don't end up dissapointed. Once you find a few restaurants or places to eat that you love and trust, you usually stick to them. The good thing is that the number of restaurants that offer GF meals is always expanding. I have also noticed more and more have it marked on their menu, which makes it even easier to order. It can be marked as GF or GFA. GFA means that a GF option is available with some simple changes. Either way always make wait staff aware that your meal **needs to be GF**, this way no mistakes will be made. Always remember if you are not sure about something, then just double check. It is a whole lot easier to double check then end up suffering later.

The main tips are

- Do some research
- Ask questions
- Make people aware of your needs
- Plan and prepare
- Eat prior to functions
- Pack some snacks

OTHER HANDY RESOURCES

At one time or another I have used these places to check on some information or as motivation and inspiration.

Coeliac Australia – www.coeliac.org.au/

Here you will find lots of helpful information about Coeliac Disease, you can find your local office and event information run by this organisation.

Australian Gluten-Free Life Magazine – a great source of information, inspiration and a great way to feel part of a community and read about what others are doing in this area. Also lots of great recipes every month, with an allergen index. Making it much easier when there are multiple food sensitivities or allergies.

Taste-Website-you can search recipes by gluten free. I have found a lot of their recipes really do turn out well.

Gluten free lunchboxes – www.glutenfreelunchboxes.com . Great ideas for kids and adult lunch boxes.

Gluten free on a shoestring – www.glutenfreeonashoestring.com . Nicole Hunn has spent more than 10 years cooking and baking gluten free. Since her son was diagnosed with Coeliac Disease she has been dedicated to making gluten free alternatives that are better than the original.

Taste gluten free cookbooks – I really like these cookbooks, as the recipes have been tested and really do work out.

Wheat and Gluten Free – small but handy cookbook by

Jody Vassallo , I got my copy at Diabetes SA.

If you believe you may have SIBO you can find more information at www.sibotest.com

Here you will find information about symptoms, the testing available and also do a quick questionnaire to see if this is a likely cause of your symptoms. You can also find health practitioners that can help with SIBO if you do test positive, like myself.

Instagram – search for gluten free and you will find heaps of people to follow and tons of inspiration.

Chapter 12

RECIPES

The recipes I have included are not ones that you would eat everyday. Just because something is GF does not mean it is healthy for you. The recipes I have included are here because these are the ones that make my husband happy when I make them. Some of them are things my husband really missed, so I have made GF versions of. For example the lasagnia is my husband's favourite meal but I only make it on special occasions.

I hope you find joy and yummyness in these recipes!

DATE AND WALNUT LOAF

YOU WILL NEED

- 1 cup chopped seedless dates
- 3 tbsp soft butter
- ½ cup coconut sugar or stevia or xylitol
- 1 Cup of water

- ½ tsp bicarb soda
- ½ tsp ground cinnamon
- 1 egg, lightly beaten
- ½ cup chopped walnuts (or any other nut you like)
- 2 cups gluten free self raising flour

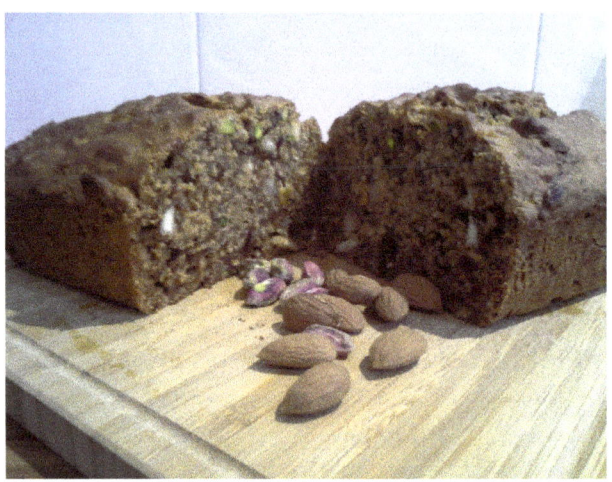

THE HOW TO

1. Line and grease a bread loaf tin with baking paper.
2. Combine dates, butter, sugar and water in a pot, stir over low heat until sugar has dissolved.
3. Bring to the boil, remove from heat and stir in the bicarb soda.
4. Let cool slightly, then stir in the cinnamon, egg, nuts and flour until well combined.

5. Pour into the bread loaf tin and bake at 170 degrees celsius in the oven for approximately 40 mins.

6. Turn n to a cooling rack and cool for 10 mins.

7. Serve sliced with a little butter.

CREPES

YOU WILL NEED

- ½ cup gluten free flour (I use FREE FROM gluten free flour – from Woolworths)
- 1 tsp rice malt syrup
- 20g butter melted
- 2 eggs
- ¾ cup full cream milk

WHAT TO DO

1. MIX rice malt syrup, butter, eggs and milk together in a small bowl
2. ADD slowly to flour in a larger bowl, whisking well with a hand whisk to get a smooth consistency.
3. POUR about 3-4 tbsp worth of mixture into a greased pan (I use a little butter) and tilt and rotate pan so the base is completely covered in mixture
4. COOK till it bubbles through and then flip over
5. CREPES should be thin, and slightly golden

PANCAKES

YOU WILL NEED

- 1 egg
- 1 ¼ cup full cream milk
- ½ cup gluten free plain flour (I use FREE FROM gluten free flour – from Woolworths)
- ½ cup gluten free self raising flour
- ¼ tsp rice malt syrup or sugar
- 2 tsp butter melted

WHAT TO DO

1. Combine the egg and milk.
2. Mix the flours and sugar, mix into the wet mixture.
3. Then beat in the melted butter with a hand whisk. Beat well until well combined and smooth.
4. Then fry in a hot pan to your desired size. Turn over when bubbles appear on the upper side.
5. Serve with your favourite toppings.

SHORTCRUST PASTRY
(can be made sweet or savoury)

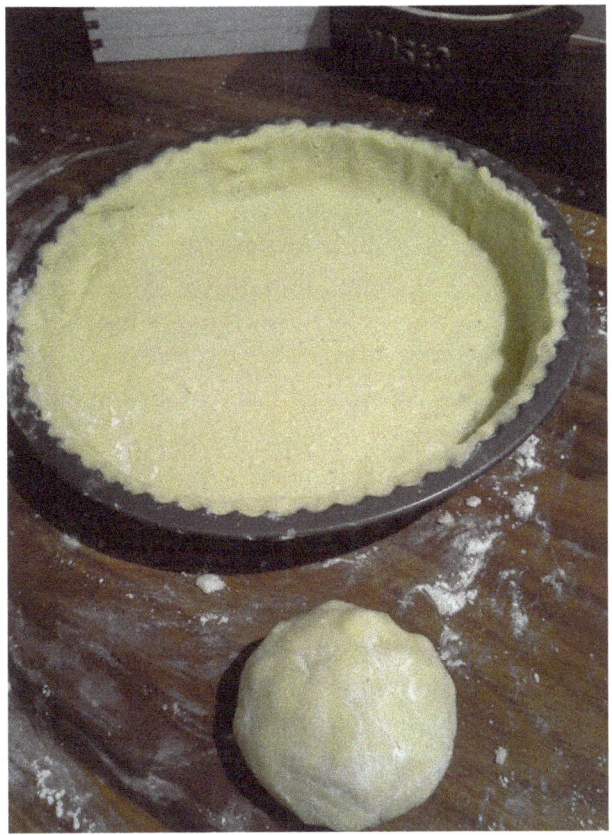

YOU WILL NEED

- 2 cups of gluten free flour (I use FREE FROM gluten free flour – from Woolworths)

- 1 tsp fine salt

- ¼ tsp gluten free baking powder

- 2 tsp tapioca flour
- 175g unsalted butter, chilled and diced
- 2 eggwhites

WHAT TO DO

1. Grease a loose bottom tart tin with butter or oil spray.
2. Sift flours, salt and baking powder into a food processor. Add diced butter, then pulse until it resembles a fine breadcrumb. Do not go too far.
3. Take out the blades, add eggwhites and start to bring it together very gently with tips of fingers to form a soft dough. If needed, you can add a touch of water. It is very important at this point not to overwork the dough.
4. Turn out the dough onto a floured bench and form into a disk. Chill in the fridge for at least an hour.
5. Roll out pastry on some floured baking paper till it is big enough for your tin. Place into the tin and remove excess from the edges. Prick the pastry with a fork. Place baking paper over the pastry and add rice to blind bake at 180 degrees celsius in the oven for 20 minutes or until lightly golden.
6. (I always keep any excess pastry wrapped in the freezer for another day. You can combine many batches to have enough for a pie or a few small ones.)
7. Note if you would like to make a sweet pie, add 2 tbsp of sugar or rice malt syrup to the pastry mixture.

TUNA, MINT AND ASPARAGUS PIE FILLING

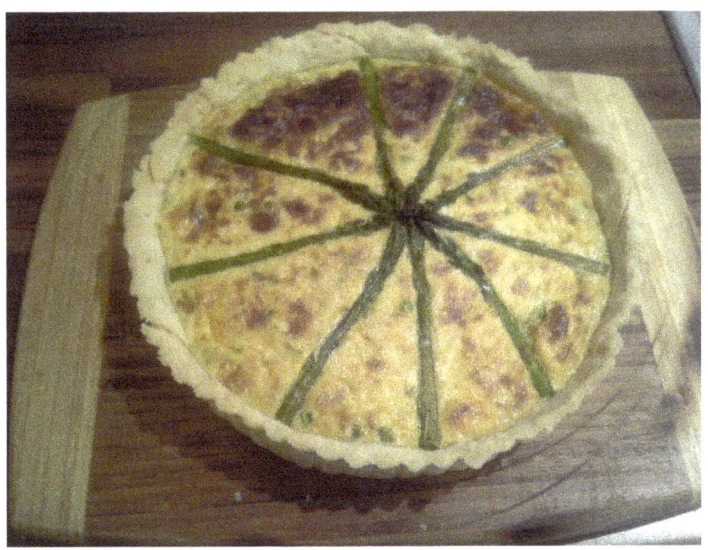

YOU WILL NEED

- 185g tin of tuna
- 150g of frozen peas
- 1 bunch of asparagus
- 3 eggs or if you are making the pastry use 2 egg yolks and 1 egg
- ¼ cup parmesan
- Handful of chopped mint leaves
- 1 tbsp Dijon mustard

- 1 ½ cups of cream <u>OR</u> 1 ½ cups of coconut cream

WHAT TO DO

1. Cut enough of the tops of the asparagus off, so that they can be fanned around the top of the pie.
2. Chop the rest of stalks into 1 cm long pieces. Combine with all the other ingredients in a bowl.
3. Pour into the pastry shell and then lay the asparagus on top of the pie.
4. Bake at 160 degrees celsius in the oven for 30 minutes or until set and golden brown.
5. Remove from the oven and let sit for 5 minutes before serving.

LASAGNE

YOU WILL NEED

MEAT SAUCE

- 1 Brown onion diced
- 8 button mushrooms sliced
- 2 rashers of bacon diced
- 500g lean beef mince
- 420g tin of diced tomato
- 420g tin of salt reduced condensed tomato soup

- ¼ cup red wine
- ½ cup stock

CHEESE SAUCE

- 60g butter
- ½ cup plain flour
- Salt and pepper
- Pinch of nutmeg
- 2 cups of milk
- 90 g grated cheddar cheese
- 2 tbsp grated parmesan cheese
- 1 box of gluten free lasagne sheets (I like to use San Remo)

WHAT TO DO

MEAT SAUCE

1. Fry the onion, mushroom and bacon in a little oil, till softened. Then add the beef and fry until mostly cooked through.
2. Then add all the liquids and simmer away till sauce thickens and looks nice and rich, probably about 30-40 minutes.

CHEESE SAUCE

1. Melt butter in a saucepan, then add the flour slowly while whisking to make it smooth. Add the salt, pepper and nutmeg. Stir over the heat for another 30 seconds.

2. Gradually add the milk, while stirring with the whisk. Once all milk is added, cook until it boils and thickens and reduce heat. Cook for a further minute.

3. Remove from heat and stir in the grated cheeses. Use the whisk to make the sauce smooth and creamy.

ASSEMBLY

1. Line the bottom of a oven proof dish with a layer of lasagne sheets. The dish I use is 18cm x 26cm.

2. Then cover a layer of meat sauce. Then cover with a thin layer of cheese sauce.

3. Repeat these three layers, 2 more times.

4. Cover with alfoil, but try to make sure it doesn't touch the top layer of cheese sauce.

5. Bake in a moderate oven for 40-60 minutes. Uncover the lasagne for the last 15 minutes so it can become golden on top.

6. Remove from the oven and let stand for 10 minutes before serving with a side salad.

EMERGENCY GF BREAD
(we make ours in a waffle press)

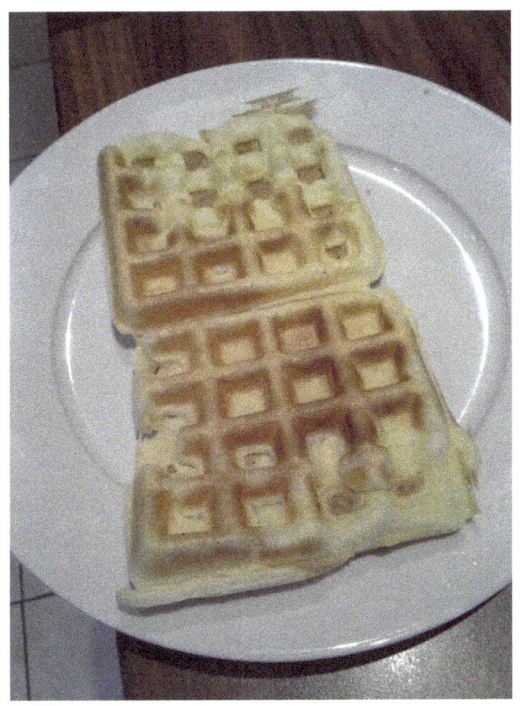

YOU WILL NEED

- 1 egg
- 1 tsp water
- 1/3 cup gluten free plain flour (I use FREE FROM gluten free flour – from Woolworths)
- ¼ tsp baking powder

- 1 tsp rice malt syrup or sugar
- 3 tbsp milk
- ¾ tsp vinegar

WHAT TO DO

1. Combine the egg, milk, vinegar.
2. Mix all the remaining ingredients into the wet mix.
3. Either pour the mix into a sandwhich plastic container and cook in the microwave (no lid) for 90seconds. Times can vary depending on your microwave. Remove from container and allow to cool. Then slice into two and toast.

OR

If you have a waffle machine, pour the mixture evenly onto the two sides of the press and cook like you would waffles. We find this gives a much nicer texture and taste.

GF FLATBREAD

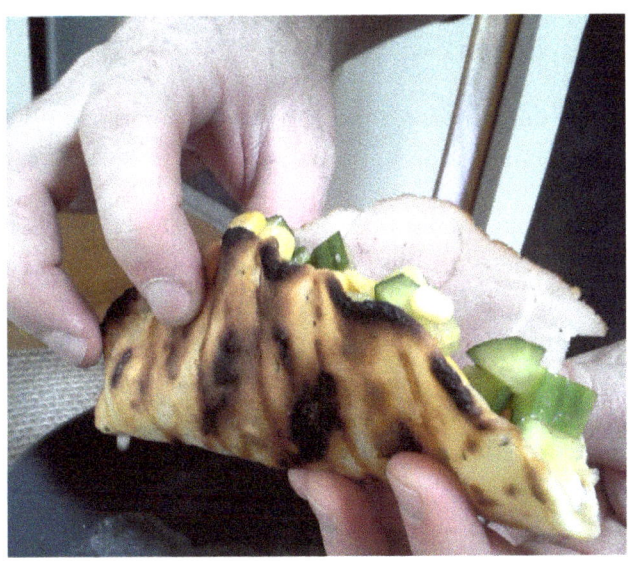

YOU WILL NEED

- 1 cup of natural yoghurt
- 1 cup of GF plain flour
- 1tbsp of olive oil
- Finely chopped rosemary and garlic to flavour the bread

WHAT TO DO

1. Place flour in a bowl, make a well in the centre and

add yoghurt and oil.

2. Combine to form a dough. If it seems too dry or wet adjust with a little more yoghurt or flour. Add the garlic and rosemary.

3. Knead gently until dough comes together and is easy to work with.

4. Divide the dough into four even portions and roll into balls.

5. Using a tortilla press (or alternatively you could place between two sheets of baking paper and use a rolling pin) Roll or press dough into circles about 0.5cm thick.

6. For best results – lightly oil or grease the dough before cooking on a BBQ grill for 3-5 minutes on each side.

CHOCOLATE COFFEE CAKE

YOU WILL NEED

CRUMBLE

- 70g grated cold butter
- 80g brown sugar
- 70g gluten free plain flour

CAKE BATTER

- 175 g melted butter

- 160g sugar, xylitol or rice malt syrup
- 3 eggs
- 70g sour cream
- 1tsp vanilla extract
- 110g hazelnut or almond meal
- 120g plain flour
- ½ tsp baking powder
- ½ cup good quality coffee
- PLUS a small bag of choc chips for sprinkling

WHAT TO DO

1. Line and grease a loose bottom spring round cake tin.
2. To make the crumble rub all the ingredients together with your fingers. Working quickly so as not to melt the butter too much. Set aside.
3. To make the batter combine the butter, sugar, eggs, sour cream and vanilla extract and mix well.
4. Then add the nut meal, flour and baking powder and combine until smooth.
5. Lastly add the coffee and stir well.
6. Now take the tin and add half the batter in an even layer. Then sprinkle half the crumble over the top, followed by half the choc chips. Then repeat these

layers again to use up the last of the mixtures.
7. Place in a preheated oven at 160 degrees celsius and bake until golden and a skewer comes out mostly clean.
8. Please note, when I bake with GF flour, I usually allow the stick to come out a little wetter than when cooking with wheat flour. This is because I have found the cake to be too dry and crumbly if I go too far. I prefer to leave a bit of moisture.

BREADCRUMBS
(don't ever waste the ends of GF bread again!)

YOU WILL NEED

- 20 ends of your gluten free bread (does not matter if they are from different styles)
- 1 garlic clove
- ¼ cup grated parmesan cheese
- 5 springs of parsley or any herb you love
- Salt & pepper

WHAT TO DO

1. I hate wasting food, so I have a bag in the freezer where I pop any ends from my husband's loaves of bread. When I have enough, (I wait for about 20 slices) I pull them out and defrost them. Then I tear them into about 6 pieces and lay them on a lined baking tray and bake them in a low oven till

they are dry and crispy.

2. Then I pull them out and let them cool. This makes sure they will be dry and crispy enough to process well in a food processor.

3. I then add some bread and the rest of the ingredients and process until I am happy with the texture. Take out and set aside in a large bowl.

4. Store in a zip lock bag in the freezer until required.

FISHCAKES

YOU WILL NEED

- 4 medium potatoes (about 600g)
- 185g tin of tuna in spring water
- ¼ cup breadcrumbs (from previous recipe)
- ¾ cup plain flour
- 1 small onion finely chopped or 3 spring onions
- 1 egg beaten
- 5 springs of parsley or any herb you love finely chopped
- Salt & pepper to taste
- ½ cup breadcrumbs to coat the fishcakes in
- Oil for cooking

WHAT TO DO

1. Peel potatoes and cut into quarters, bring to boil in a medium sized pot and cook until tender. Mash and allow to cool.

2. Place the tuna, mash potato, breadcrumbs, flour and onion in a bowl. Mix well to combine. Then add the herbs, egg and salt and pepper.

3. Shape into patties, roll in the extra breadcrumbs and place on a plate. Once all are made, place in the fridge to rest and set for at least 30 minutes.

4. Heat oil and shallow fry gently till golden.

5. Serve with a salad or vegetables.

6. Remainder can be frozen for another meal.

FREE GIFT TO YOU

If you live in Adelaide or are planning to visit and would love a very comprehensive restaurant and cafe list then please email me at tummyrescue@gmail.com

Simply enter your name and GF EATS in the subject line

And I will email you a copy of my special resource so you can love every minute of eating out in our city.

CONTACT ME

If you would like to have a consult with me or have any questions please feel free to get in touch

Tummy Rescue
Website: www.tummyrescue.com.au
Email: tummyrescue@gmail.com

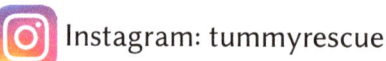 Instagram: tummyrescue

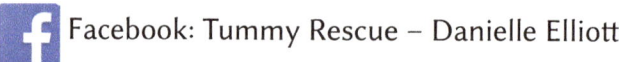 Facebook: Tummy Rescue – Danielle Elliott

Lightning Source UK Ltd.
Milton Keynes UK
UKHW020649300721
387993UK00003B/20